"Virgie Tovar is a vita[...]
ism, media, and femin[...]
own body and life, com[...]
she expresses at an opp[...], is a truly radical
act. Tovar is deeply thoughtful, but does not equivo-
cate. She confronts bigotry, but does not engage with
bullshit."

> —**KELSEY MILLER, author of** *Big Girl:*
> *How I Gave Up Dieting and Got a Life*

"Fierce, passionate, and poignant, *You Have the Right
to Remain Fat* is a manifesto that will inspire you and
ignite the revolution."

> —**LINDA BACON, author of** *Health at Every Size:*
> *The Surprising Truth about Your Weight*

"The importance of Virgie Tovar's perspective and
identity cannot be overstated. As we collectively decon-
struct our society's addiction to body negativity, her
words provide crucial guidance, clarity, and support for
all those who champion universal body liberation."

> —**JESSAMYN STANLEY, author of** *Every Body Yoga:*
> *Let Go of Fear, Get on the Mat, Love Your Body*

"Lucid, joyous, mad as hell, and making a whole lot of
sense."

> —**JOANNA WALSH, author of**
> *Worlds from the Word's End*

"In this era of so-called 'body positivity,' Virgie Tovar
is the radical voice we need. One of our best writers on
fat and a leading figure in fat activism, she has a gift
for expressing what so many women feel but cannot
always articulate. In this bold new book, Tovar evisccr-
ates diet culture, proclaims the joyous possibilities of
fatness, and shows us that liberation is possible."

> —**SARAI WALKER, author of** *Dietland*

"Virgie Tovar has authored a fantastic book that is witty, warm, and wise. You want to gobble up her words, she shows how powerful and political personal writing can be. Full of energy and spark."

—CHARLOTTE COOPER, author of
Fat Activism: A Radical Social Movement

"*You Have the Right to Remain Fat* feels like spending a margarita-soaked day at the beach with your smartest friend. Virgie Tovar shares juicy secrets and makes revolutionary ideas viscerally accessible. You'll be left enlightened, inspired, happier, and possibly angrier than when you started."

—JOY NASH, actress

"Virgie Tovar does the thing we need to see more of in political writing: she shares every bit of her humanity. Her clear descriptions of anti-fat bias and the social construction that is 'diet culture' make it difficult to disagree with her main point: *you* are not the problem, *society* is the problem. The world desperately needs to be told this truth."

—ISABEL FOXEN DUKE, creator of
StopFightingFood.com

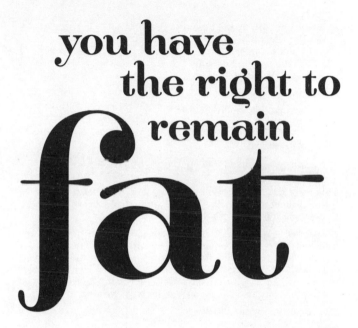

you have the right to remain fat

VIRGIE TOVAR

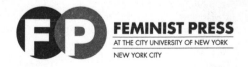

FEMINIST PRESS
AT THE CITY UNIVERSITY OF NEW YORK
NEW YORK CITY

Published in 2018 by the Feminist Press
at the City University of New York
The Graduate Center
365 Fifth Avenue, Suite 5406
New York, NY 10016

feministpress.org

First Feminist Press edition 2018

NEW YORK STATE OF OPPORTUNITY. | Council on the Arts

This book was made possible thanks to a grant from New York State Council on the Arts with the support of Governor Andrew Cuomo and the New York State Legislature.

First printing August 2018

Edited by Michelle Tea

Cover and text design by Drew Stevens

Library of Congress Cataloging-in-Publication Data
Names: Tovar, Virgie, 1982- author.
Title: You have the right to remain fat / Virgie Tovar.
Description: New York, NY : Feminist Press, 2018. | Includes bibliographical references.
Identifiers: LCCN 2017049772 (print) | LCCN 2017053575 (ebook) | ISBN 9781936932320 (e-book) | ISBN 9781936932313 (trade pbk.)
Subjects: LCSH: Overweight women. | Body image in women. | Self-esteem in women. | Discrimination against overweight persons.
Classification: LCC RC628 (ebook) | LCC RC628 .T683 2018 (print) | DDC
613/.04244—dc23
LC record available at https://lccn.loc.gov/2017049772

Contents

Introduction

My body used to belong to me.

When I was a little girl, my favorite part of the day was when we got home from errands or preschool. I would push the front door open with both small hands and run—through the living room filled with plastic-wrapped furniture, past the washer dryer that made funny sounds that I liked, past my bedroom filled with a growing collection of Winnie the Pooh toys—into the bathroom. I would take all my clothes off as quickly as possible, shimmying out of my underwear and pants, breaking out of my shirt like it was an inconvenient membrane. I would leave the pile on the floor and then run back out, giggling with uncontained delight, to the kitchen where my grandmother was always cooking.

I would stop at the end of the little hall, where the calico-cat-colored rug met the linoleum of the dining room. I would spread out my arms and legs as far as I could. And I would jiggle. My thighs and belly, my cheeks and my whole body would wobble. I would turn my head in circles. I liked that everything moved and undulated. My body was like the water in the bathtub or the water at the community pool, which I loved so much in the summer. My body was like that water, a source of relief and fun, a place I could jump into and be held. It felt good. Oh, it felt so good. I remember how curious I was, and how much I loved that my body could do these incredible things. I had no sense of self-awareness, only the immediacy of pleasure.

I think back on that time in my life as if it was someone else's story. It feels so far away. I feel protective of that little girl, who couldn't imagine the horrible education awaiting her.

Less than a year later, those jiggle-filled afternoons would disappear. I would find myself being taught by boys at school that I was unlovable and disgusting because of my fat body. I would lose sight of how magical my body was, how magical I was. I would lose the sense that my body was mine at all.

All the freedom and wonder I felt became supplanted by a sharp sense that I had failed at something big. And that it was my job to fix it—to fix me. Rather than learning to trust my instincts and value myself, I learned that the size of my body was the only thing that mattered about me.

Through a series of violent, culturally sanctioned events—so commonplace that women simply call them "life"—my innate relationship to my body was taken from me and replaced with something foreign and alien and harmful. My relationship to my body was replaced with one toxic idea: your body is wrong. This idea would threaten my happiness and my health for nearly two decades.

As much as I wish it were, my story is not unique. It is, in many ways, the story of women's lives in America.

As I was writing the introduction to this book, I got an email from a woman who told me that she was being treated for bulimia, an eating disorder that disproportionately affects women and only exists in cultures that glorify thinness. Even though she was seeking treatment for a disorder that threatened her very life, she was still cautioned against gaining "too much" weight while in recovery. Her email reminded me of the first time I'd heard such a story. A woman told me she had cancer that went untreated because her doctor told her that the problem was her weight. She went in for an appointment because she was experiencing excruciating menstrual cramps and very heavy periods. She was afraid. Rather than examining her, the doctor told her that if she lost weight that everything would be fine. Had the doctor been willing to take her seriously, she could have found the lump in her uterus, but instead it grew unchecked for another three years. And I was reminded of my own childhood and my education in body shame that sought to steal from me the most precious thing I would ever have: the inherent magic of being alive *and* the vehicle through which that magic is experienced, my body.

The perpetrators of these stories are body shame, fatphobia, and dieting, which hide behind the seemingly innocuous language of "self-improvement," "inspiration," and "health." In many ways, however, these ideas are merely symptoms of a larger cultural problem, not least our country's history of unresolved racism, white supremacy, classism, and misogyny.

While we have spent the last twenty-five years cleaning up the sexist residue in our vocabulary, we have been living out woman-hating methods of control via our dinner plates and our bathroom scales—often not even knowing that this is what we are doing. We are giving away our lives, our time, our energy, our claim to pleasure, our desire, and our power one bite at a time. Submission has taken on a new face: where once there was barred access to meaningful employment and the right to vote, sexism today has morphed into skipped meals and too many hours spent at the gym. As Naomi Wolf famously wrote in *The Beauty Myth*, "Dieting is the most potent political sedative in women's history."

I promise you that everything I tell you here is the truth, as well as I can tell it, of my seven years spent researching diet culture and fatphobia. I promise you that I don't have an agenda besides my deepest desire that reading this book will leave you with some tools to combat this horrible assisted femicide masked as diet culture. I will admit that I want you to get super pissed off that you have been lied to and that there are cultural forces actively attempting to dismantle the most precious parts of your selfhood right now—and then getting you to pay for that violent process. It is only when we stop lying to ourselves that we can stop being lied to by others. It is only when we trust our own experience of the truth that we can be free.

Diet culture seeks to undermine that very thing: self-trust—our inner compass, that reptilian and prehistoric guide living inside us, our greatest inheritance accumulated over generations of living on this planet.

And that's why I wrote this book. I write from a place of professional and personal investment. Professionally I am a body-image expert, lecturer, and author, as well as a scholar in the emerging discipline of fat studies. Personally I am a fatshionista, a vociferous activist, a lover of creamy pastries, a world traveler, a potty mouth, and a San Francisco bohemian who loves pedicures, cheetah print, and Chihuahuas, and who couldn't live without mimosas, huge sunglasses, tiny bathing suits, and my Hitachi Magic Wand. I am also a 250-pound woman who chose to stop dieting because I wanted to start living my life rather than continue dreaming about it.

I used to believe that I was afraid of food and of being fat, but now I know that the fear was of a deeply troubled culture that would not allow me to thrive. A culture that was, in fact, invested in my degradation.

It is with great urgency that I write to women directly. Whatever I tell you in the following pages is told with the greatest desire to see women live the life we all deserve to live—the life that our wider culture will never grant you, the one that you must take. The key to that life is the unbridling of our desire. This culture teaches us to extinguish that desire the moment we are taught that women shouldn't be fat. I say, you have the right to remain fat.

What Are Fatphobia and Diet Culture?

I think it's almost a fact that everyone remembers that kid in their class who used to look up all the girls' skirts. For me, that person was Joshua. Preschool. We were four. I remember one day we had been crawling around in a brightly colored plastic tube, like one of those gerbil mazes for toddlers. I was breathless from trying to escape him. I was mostly pretending he was chasing me; he was actually chasing a smaller girl who was behind me in the gerbil tube. He always chased and terrorized girls, trying to look up their skirts. He never tried to look up mine, though, and I sensed that his rejection augured something bigger.

I don't think it's a coincidence that the boy who looked up skirts was also the first person who ever called me fat. Or at least the first person I remember calling me that. After all, unsolicited masculine sexual attention and the drive to control feminine bodies go hand in hand.

I remember we were both standing on the blacktop, and that's when he said it. "You're fat."

I was confused. I didn't have any context for the word. It wasn't a word that had been in my world before then, but there was something about the way he said it. I could tell from the way he hurled it out of his mouth, like snot, that it was a hurtful word, a word meant to remind me that I had forgotten something about who I was.

I knew there was some distant connection between my wish for him to look up my skirt and his desire to hurt me.

I just stared at him, trying to calculate this new reality. It wouldn't be long before I was in kindergarten and I would hear that word all the time. I would become that word, and I would adopt that hatred toward myself that my classmates had for me.

For a long time, I didn't know that other people's hatred wasn't my fault, and I didn't know that their hatred had a name. Fatphobia is a form of bigotry that positions fat people as inferior and as objects of hatred and derision. Fatphobia targets and scapegoats fat people, but it ends up harming all people. Everyone ends up in one of two camps: they are either living the pointed reality of fatphobic bigotry or they are living in fear of becoming subject to it. So, fatphobia uses the treatment of fat people as a means of controlling the body size of all people. Fatphobia creates an environment of hostility toward large-bodied people, promotes a pathological relationship to food and movement (which, when dieting, transforms into diet and exercise), and places the burden of anti-fat bias on "noncompliant" individuals—that is, fat people.

Because of the way fat people are positioned in our culture, people learn to fear becoming fat. They are afraid of discrimination and hatred. It is *normal* to feel afraid of people hating you. It is *not* normal for people to hate anyone based on how much they weigh. It is furthermore not normal, fair, or ethical to feel you have to comply with body-conformity expectations in order to avoid hatred and discrimination. We as a culture have characterized being fat as an inherently bad thing, when in reality body size is meaningless and lacks the good or bad associations imposed by wider culture. We were not born thinking fat is bad and thin is good. We learn these things through an ongoing cultural education.

In no example did this become clearer to me than when I began reading the work of anthropologists doing ethnographies in regions of the contemporary world where women go to extreme lengths to be as fat as possible. I will return to this research later on.

When we take a moment to recognize what our culture teaches us about fat people, it becomes really clear really quickly that fatphobia is a form of bigotry, obscured by the naturalizing language of beauty and health and the false narrative of concern.

A recent experience that cemented the reality of fatphobic bigotry in my mind happened when I was attending a conference for fat queers called NOLOSE. Unlike previous years, the conference was held in Portland, Oregon, rather than Oakland, California, and was at a much larger hotel than ever before. For the first time, we were sharing accommodations with many other guests who were not associated with the conference. In Oakland, we take over the hotel.

Over the course of the three-day conference, we were gawked at like oddities because
almost all of the conference participants were
fat. The pool was near the lobby and people would line up, noses pressed against the
glass, to stare at us while we were swimming.
Several participants were followed and intim-
idated by guests from our hotel and even a
neighboring one. Some of these guests even
forced their way into private events and
refused to leave despite requests from conference volunteers and hotel staff. At one point,
I was waiting for an elevator and as the doors
opened I heard a man say, "There's one of
them!" speaking to a group of two women and
two children, and pointing at me. He was following conference attendees around with his
family offering commentary like he was leading a tour in a zoo. I finally approached him
and his family in the middle of a hotel hall-
way. I clocked them entering their room from
about three hundred feet away, and my anger
was unleashed. I told him how disgusting
it was that he was behaving like a bigot in
front of his family. I didn't see him again for
the remainder of the weekend. Thank Saint
Stevie Nicks (if we're going to invoke a deity

let it be Stevie). It's important to instill the fear of the unhinged fat feminist into shameless fatphobes.

After that ugly encounter, some of my fat friends and I decided to get lunch. We decided that the hotel restaurant would be easy, and so the six of us filed in and sat down. The menus were on the table, and after a few minutes the waitress came over. She greeted us by saying (no joke), "Let me guess, you people all want separate checks." I was legitimately shocked by her hateful language. *You people?* She stood with her hip cocked and an air of uncontained annoyance at our audacity for having come into the restaurant of the hotel where we were all staying. A hush overtook the entire table. The women I was with lowered their heads, and one after the other they offered their orders quietly and apologetically. This woman had triggered them. She had reminded all of us of moments throughout our lives when fatphobes had talked to us as if they wished we didn't exist, as if we were less than others. When it came time for me to tell her what I was having, I refused to order anything and instead asked, "Is there any reason you are treating everyone at this table so unacceptably?"

In that moment, something bizarre happened. She paused for a second, her face frozen, and then completely snapped out of bigotry mode and into sweet-as-pie mode. It was like watching a robot switch programs from asshole to artifice in two seconds flat. She didn't apologize, but from that moment forward she didn't snap out of her customer-service mode again. We decided that the way we wanted to deal with the situation was to finish the meal and not leave a tip. Someone recently introduced me to the concept of "radical pettiness," and I feel like this was one of those moments where all we could do was fight bigotry with a small capitalist retaliation. I'd never experienced fatphobia in a collective way before. When I'm alone I am easy to dismiss, but when I'm part of a group of fat people, my existence creates a sense of threat that needs to be squashed. That day I felt like we were not only being socially punished for being fat but for liking ourselves enough that we would be seen with others who looked like us.

In our culture, fat people are used to scapegoat anxieties about excess, immorality, and an uncontained relationship to desire and consumption. Most people are raised to believe myriad bigoted beliefs about fat inferiority and see this fictional creation as a natural truth. They don't see these beliefs as political, cultural, or particularly problematic. They often don't even totally know they have these feelings. They just see fatphobia as part of life, the way that oxygen or clouds are just part of life. The culture puts a lot of energy into forcing people to stay in that sad place of unquestioned fatphobia.

Dieting is a practice of fatphobia.

Dieting is the result of unresolved fatphobia. We become terrified of what it would mean for us to be fat because we understand fundamentally how poorly fat people are treated. We transpose that bigotry onto the fat itself, rather than placing the blame where it belongs: on the culture that created and promotes injustice and fat hatred. We thereby, perhaps unintentionally, end up blaming fat people for the bigotry they are experiencing. Even though fatphobia is culturally pervasive and treated as if it's a totally normal part of everyday life, it's important to recognize that it is a form of bigotry that really harms people and that must be eradicated.

The concomitant rise of body positivity, plus-size fashion, and fitness-app usage has led to the near extinction of the term "dieting." In its wake, a flurry of new, more specific, and more dynamic language has arisen. It's the process of transmuting a diet (i.e., restricting calories) to "taking care of one's health."

For example, juicing—essentially a diet—is not a new concept. In the eighties, its benefits were boiled down entirely to weight loss. But today rather than calling it a "juice diet" or "liquid diet," it's simply called "juicing," bringing the term out of the explicit realm of weight loss and into a gray area where the goal of weight loss becomes unclear or plausibly deniable. However, if juicing were believed to have incredible health benefits but led to weight gain, it would lose all its appeal for women.

Though the word "diet" has gone out of vogue, what remains are all the mechanisms and ideologies of dieting—all the things I've outlined above—but the language is just harder to understand. The language used to sell diet products has shifted away from shame and fear in favor of aspiration and optimization. Rather than specifically focusing on weight loss, there are more references to "health" and the idea that "healthy is the new skinny." But know this: any lifestyle or plan or philosophy or app that treats weight loss as a goal is a diet. Anything that would lose appeal if didn't lead to the acquisition or maintenance of a thin(ner) body is a diet. Period.

I often ask people, can you imagine going one single day without hearing about calories, without someone referring to potato chips as evil, without worrying for a second about how much fat is in something, or without wishing that you were thinner? Most people answer no.

And that is what transforms dieting as an individual behavior into diet culture: its unavoidability, the way it seeps imperceptibly into thoughts and worldviews and interactions, the fact that people can't opt out of it. Right now, even though I know how violent and absurd and unnecessary diet culture is, I can't even imagine a world beyond it most of the time. And I'm a super-hopeful fat-positive feminist who refuses to diet and wears crop tops and Miss Piggy jewelry.

Diet culture is the marriage of the multi-billion-dollar diet industry (including fitness apps, over-the-counter diet pills, prescription drugs to suppress appetite, bariatric surgery, gyms, and gym clothiers) and the social and cultural atmosphere that normalizes weight control and fatphobic bigotry.

We cannot honestly discuss diet culture without recognizing that fatphobia and diet culture go together like milk and cookies. Many women never make this connection, believing they are not thin enough because they have food addictions or unresolved trauma, but often what is at the core of their anxiety is actually being fat. We must axiomatically reject the idea that fatness is only ever a product of trauma, mental illness, or imbalance. This narrative is false. We must name the truth in order to free ourselves from the fears that have burrowed into our psyches.

Restriction Doesn't Work: It's Not You

For nearly twenty years I was on a diet. I was restricting what I ate and trying to manipulate my body shape and size through exercise. Every single bite of food felt like a grand drama being played out on the stage of my life. Every day began with a sense of disappointment. I felt like I had failed myself, Richard Simmons, and the whole wide world. I read articles about "easy" diet tips in my grandma's copies of *Woman's World*. I listened to interviews with "fitness gurus." I ate grapefruit. So much grapefruit. I watched Susan Powter's *Stop the Insanity!* with the same religiosity that many people watch televangelists. Dieting was my religion, and my salvation was always just around the corner.

My weight frequently fluctuated, but not by much. No matter what happened, though, I never blamed diets. I never blamed Susan

Powter. I never blamed *Woman's World.* I didn't blame grapefruit. I blamed myself. It never occurred to me that the diet industry was lying to me and everyone else. That it was relying on the knowledge that women blame ourselves for how we are treated. The diet industry was using language like "easy" and "simple" to manipulate dieters everywhere into believing that if their programs didn't work it was because we were using them incorrectly.

Here's a fact: despite all the promises of the diet industry, paradoxically, dieting leads to weight gain over time. Let me say that again: over time, dieting leads to weight gain. I say there's nothing wrong with weight gain, but the culture says differently. So, if the stated goal of thinness is not actually being achieved, then what are we *really* doing when we are dieting?

Dieting doesn't do the thing it's allegedly designed to do, but dieting does lead to a number of other results: low self-esteem and decreased self-advocacy during sexual nego-tiation (there is some evidence that suggests that fat women negotiate for condoms less frequently than their thin counterparts[1]). Fat people experience more anxiety in our daily lives. We experience the effects of something called "minority stress"—the negative physiological outcomes of discrimination, cruelty, and social ostracization over a lifetime.[2] That stress can result in suppressed immunity, shortened life span, and decreased heart health—not coincidentally, some of the very things often attributed to high body weight in the medical industry. Further, if we all miraculously became our doctor-recommended BMI overnight, we would awake the following day to find that the goal post had been moved because control is the ultimate purpose of diet culture and fatphobia.

What is the alternative? To stop. Stop being terrified of fatness. Stop marginalizing fat people. To recognize that no body is superior or inferior to another. My core belief is both painfully obvious and wholly subversive: every person, regardless of weight or health status, deserves to live a life completely free from bigotry and discrimination.

That might sound really simple, but imagine for one second what this really means: that *you* would have full access to all the things that matter most to you no matter how big or small *you* are, whether you were able to run a mile in eight minutes or you hadn't run a day in your life. No caveats, no fine print— just you and your life, without any barriers you perceive to be in your way due to weight or body shape.

This means you wouldn't feel the need to change your body size in order to be taken seriously as a romantic partner. You wouldn't internalize your body's limits as a personal failure because you would have no framework for your body as a source of failure.

This means that you would not be socially punished if you gained forty pounds and you would not be socially rewarded if you lost forty pounds. (I believe there would likely be significantly less weight fluctuation without diet culture and fatphobia.)

This means that when you went to the doctor you wouldn't be treated differently or be refused proper treatment if you were fat.

This means that food would be stripped of moral meaning, which would make eating less terrifying. You wouldn't feel morally inferior if you ate tacos rather than a salad since food shame wouldn't be a thing.

This means that when you had important

moments in your life you wouldn't be expected to lose a bunch of weight. So you could focus on the joy of those important moments rather than being distracted by anxiety.

This means that the idea of sweating all over your clothes in a public space filled with fitness machinery solely to lose weight would not make you feel like you were becoming a "better person."

This means that the gym industry's current business model—which actually relies upon members signing up in January and then not ever using the gym (really!)—wouldn't work.[3]

You wouldn't feel compelled to talk about how potato chips are "evil." Your coworkers wouldn't haggle over the tiniest sliver of birthday cake. (You know that one person who says "a little smaller" on repeat.) You wouldn't break out in a cold sweat every time you walked past ice cream at the grocery store. And we wouldn't be handing over sixty billion dollars a year to the diet industry.

This means that when you thought of how you would look in the future, you would be the same size in your fantasies as you are right now.

This means that you would stop actively

trying to control your weight and just focus on other stuff—like your life, what and who makes you happy, and the pursuits that matter to you.

You can begin to see the ways fatphobia manifests in not just the obvious avoidance of weight gain but also in the way we imagine important moments and our future selves. It's kind of scary to think of all that because then you have to admit just how pervasive size-based bigotry and fatphobia really are.

Dieting: Family, Assimilation, and Bootstrapping

I grew up a self-assured, bossy, ridiculous, theatrical little fat girl. If I wanted to do an impromptu forty-five-minute talent show featuring only me in the middle of dinner, this was viewed as totally normal, and actually quite laudable, behavior. I was always eccentric. My mom, grandma, and grandpa are all very fashionable people. My mother used to be a master thrifter, often purchasing things like denim skirts and overalls from the second-hand store down the street, cutting them into mini versions of their original manifestations, and then adding lace flourishes and puffy paint to create elaborate rococo ensembles. My grandmother is a bit more reserved but loves a good sparkly flourish. In her old age, she has developed an affinity for glitter nail polish from Daiso. My grandfather was a peacock—always dressed in yellows, greens, hot pinks, sometimes even in floral prints. He had gold teeth and a 1993 gold Ford Thunderbird to match, which I inherited after he passed away in 2015.

My family isn't perfect. In fact, my family is highly dysfunctional, but they have always been very good at making me feel like the queen of the world. I grew up feeling worshipped in a lot of ways. In fact, my pet name in childhood was *reina*, the Spanish word for "queen."

My grandparents raised me, and they were both immigrants from Mexico. I grew up learning osmotically how to code-switch, hustle, make a dollar out of fifteen cents, and love America: Capitalism. Sandwiches. Cap'n Crunch. Rainbow Brite. She-Ra. Peanut butter. Barbie. Fruit snacks. Singing songs about how anyone could grow up to be president.

Bootstrapping was something I watched my family do proudly every day of my life. The idea behind bootstrapping is that anyone can earn anything as long as they want it badly enough; all they have to do is pull themselves up by their bootstraps. This is one of the primary cornerstones of American aesthetics and ideology.

It is also a foundation of diet culture.

Unlike many parts of the world where fate is considered to be something that lies beyond the reach of average humans, in the US fate is considered to be something that is resoundingly within the realm of every single person's control. Failure is an individual problem, not a collective, cultural, or political problem. The idea is that if you don't have something, it is because you didn't want it badly enough, or you didn't try hard enough. Though the allure of this idea is undeniable, there isn't much room for serious considerations of justice or historical unfairness in this narrative. But it is this fantasy—the American Dream—that is the siren song for so many. It was the siren song for me and my family.

Bootstrapping is as American as apple fucking pie.

My grandfather was a "never missed a day of work in his life" kind of man. He knew what Americans thought of Mexicans, and so he always felt the pressure to be twice as good. He always wore cologne and applied hair oil so he looked coiffed. Every night he scrubbed his fingernails with harsh detergent not meant for the delicate skin of his hands.

He spent so much time reading books, learning new English words, and always trying to outsmart everyone. He picked up every extra hour offered at his job. He saved and budgeted and went to church and bought a home. He went from being a janitor to the head chemist at the factory where he worked for twenty years. He was a "good" Mexican man. He was the evidence that anyone could start anywhere and make something of themselves. What was invisible to the outside world was how tormented he was, how much he worried, how often he cried in secret, and how ashamed he was of his sadness. He didn't speak of the times that he was humiliated or passed over because he had an accent. He was filled with rage, but he took it out on himself and the people he loved the most—my grandmother and our family.

In many ways, his story of bootstrapping was a lot like my own. I gradually learned that I was less than others because I was a fat brown girl. The lessons I learned about the inferiority of my fat body were brutal; the lessons I received about my racial and gender inferiority were subtle by comparison.

But both educations were real, and in some ways, the brutality of fatphobia made it easier for me to recognize its existence later. All I wanted was for people to treat me like a person. I thought I could bootstrap myself into humanity.

As I grew up working my little ass off to get straight As so I could go to one of the top one hundred colleges and work in an office and wear suits every day (success!), I didn't even skip a beat when I was asked to bootstrap with my weight. Dieting maps seamlessly onto the preexisting American narrative of failure and success as individual endeavors.

The way I understood it, my weight was clearly a problem—my problem. I learned that it was my responsibility to fix my problems. I wasn't taught that some people don't like fat people because they are bigots, and it's their responsibility not to be bigots. I was taught that everyone on the planet hates fat people because it is a universal and undeniable truth that fat people are bad. Presented in this way, I had no room to understand my treatment as unethical or even odd. I accepted it as the truth that had existed forever and ever. It wasn't until I began researching the history and sociology of fatness that I would learn that the way we fear fat is socially constructed. "Fat" and "thin" are make-believe categories the way "gay" and "straight" are. They were brought into existence for no other reason than to control people.

Dieting Is a Survival Technique

I went on an "extreme" diet for the first time when I was eleven years old. I had been restricting what I ate for several years before then, but this experience was different. I called it dieting, but I was actually starving myself. I did it during the summer between fifth and sixth grades because I wanted to end my final year of elementary school with a body makeover like the one I had seen in the 1989 made-for-TV movie starring Tony Danza, *She's Out of Control*.

Tony was a single dad who had a fat, nerdy daughter in high school. Her name was Katie. The movie opens up with her doing exercise in her bedroom. She's running in place wearing spandex pants. She's got glasses and braces on. She's an underdog. Then Tony's girlfriend helps her get a makeover. She goes from a nottie to a hottie once her braces and glasses are gone. After all her bedroom workouts, her fat body is also gone. She's curvy in exactly the right way—the way that gives men boners. All the boys who had ignored her or had been mean to her drool over her now. Her body had gone from a source of pity and spite to a source of jealousy and desire. I watched that movie over and over again—almost as if by watching it I could make it real for me. *She's Out of Control* was my church! I wanted to be Katie. I wanted to give everyone a boner.

I remember how important that summer was for me. It symbolized the possibility of radical transformation. My idea of fun was not swimming pools or eating popsicles, it was the idea that I could use the heat of the sun and the freedom of not attending school to commit myself entirely to becoming thin. I spent three months eating nothing but toast and lettuce. Twice a day I would put the sixty-minute step-aerobics VHS tape I had found at the thrift store into the VCR. I didn't have a Step so I would try to move my body to mirror the impact, crouching low to make my thighs work harder. I didn't lose a lot of weight, but I did change sizes very quickly.

I went to my family's doctor to show off my new body. Dr. McCole always tried to incentivize my weight loss by telling me that when I got thin he would let me date one of his sons. I used to laugh when he said that, slightly humiliated but still wanting to earn the right to make his sons love me. As I sat on the exam table he congratulated me on my lowered weight. He did not ask me how I lost the weight. He did not ask me what I was or wasn't eating. It didn't matter. Literally no one seemed to care. He believed, like most, that when a fat woman—or girl—loses weight, it's always positive no matter how the loss happened.

I went back to school, ready for my accolades. I felt so proud. I had finally done what everyone had told me to do. I had finally taken the extreme measures necessary to change. To my chagrin, I hadn't read the fine print. Sure, I had lost weight, but I hadn't lost enough. To my horror and surprise, I was still everyone's idea of fat. I was tall for my age and I had boobs. I still had my double

chin and my chubby cheeks. I wasn't frail or
waifish. I had misunderstood, or maybe the
goalpost had moved, while I was busy eating
toast and fake stepping.

I would undertake starvation again as a
freshman in college while I was living abroad.
This time my body was more broken down
from the intervening years of self-imposed
malnutrition. So it didn't take long before I
started to become ill. I lost my sense of equilib-
rium about a month and a half after I stopped
eating. I began to experience dizzy spells and
nausea. I was so exhausted from the lack of
food that I would need to sit down and rest
frequently and would often fall asleep. Once
I sat down on a public bench one block from
my apartment because I was so exhausted I
couldn't make it home. I woke up in the middle of the night, the streets empty. I was all
alone and terrified in another country I barely
knew. In fact, I almost missed my flight back
to the States because I fell asleep while I was
waiting to board the plane. I was about a hundred feet from the ticket counter. Apparently
they had been paging me on the intercom,
but I hadn't heard. When I woke up, I ran to
the door and the flight attendant gave me a

stern look, chastising me for holding up
the boarding process. I remember thinking
that she had no idea why I was so tired, and
maybe she wouldn't have been so mean to me
if she knew that I was trying my hardest to
be good.

My body did not respond to dieting the way
I thought it was supposed to. Everyone says
that it's simple: calories in, calories out. An
objective mathematical reality. That didn't
seem to be true for me. I've since learned that
it's not true for many people. At the time, I
thought my body had betrayed me. I thought I
was weak and my body was defective because
I couldn't get down to what I considered my
"ideal" size. I realize now that what I put my
body through was abusive. I was treating my
body like a thing that was worthless unless
it looked the way I thought it was supposed
to look. It took years to realize that my body
was actually doing miraculous things all the
time—the way my lungs metabolized oxygen,
the way my liver cleaned my blood, the way
my eyes could detect a million colors. When
I gave myself the space to revel in what my
body could do, I realized how much I'd under-
estimated it.

As I was thinking about the idea of writing this book, I realized how apt the word "survival" is when discussing diet culture. Dieting is itself a survival technique—a way of attempting to feel control, a way of communicating to the culture that you understand what is expected of you and are willing to act on those expectations obediently. Obedience is about the recognition that the odds are stacked against you and that giving in is your only shot.

It has been my experience that women don't diet because they want to, but because they feel they have to. The sense of obligation is a sign of distress.

Internalized Inferiority
and Sexism

In 2016, for the first time in my life, I tried to explain the connections between sexism, dieting, and internalized inferiority to a group of people. Specifically I was trying to explain that internalized inferiority is part of sexism and diet culture feeds on that sense of inferiority. I was giving a lecture about diet culture to a bunch of high school students in Menlo Park, California. Most of the young women in attendance sat in their seats, leaning forward with this expression I can only call the "someone is finally speaking some truth" face. I have noticed that when I talk about the sexism that is inherent in diet culture and fatphobia, I am simply giving language to a feeling most women already have.

So I want you to imagine me on a little stage with a podium, my PowerPoint behind me, a bunch of supersmart sixteen-year-olds before me—mainly girls, but some guys too.

I told them there was a really good chance that if I asked each of the women in the room "Do you feel inferior?" they would most likely say no. They might even scoff as if I were asking a ridiculous question. I imagine that if I asked the average American woman born after the women's liberation movement this question, she would reply in the same way.

Then I pushed them further:

"So maybe you don't consciously feel inferior, but what if I asked you some follow-up questions, like:

"Today are you wearing something that is physically uncomfortable because you believe it makes you look better?

"Today did you refuse to eat something you wanted to eat because you were worried what it might do to the way you look?

"Today did you refuse to do something you wanted to do because you were worried about how it would make you look to another person?

"Today did you deny an impulse to say no or yes to something that mattered to you because you were worried that someone wouldn't like you if you did it?"

I told the young women in the audience that if I were going to make an educated guess, I would bet that they said yes to several, if not all, of the follow-up questions. Yet all of those questions were about gauging entrenched inferiority beliefs. How could they answer no to the question of inferiority and answer yes to the questions about whether they engaged in inferiority-based behavior? I watched a number of the teachers in the audience nod in recognition. The young women seemed sort of stunned, and I was too busy giving them deep eye contact to notice how the guys were reacting, but my guess is that they were either feeling annoyed that I had revealed something that would now make their future relationships with the women in the room more difficult—or they were on Reddit. It's always complicated to have defensive men in the room when I'm unveiling the secret mechanisms of patriarchy. They often don't understand their own investment in the oppression of women because it has been so naturalized for them.

I finished the lecture with these thoughts, "Inferiority at its core can simply be described as the idea that someone or some group of people aren't good enough or worthy enough at all times without conditions or caveats. When an idea becomes part of a person's worldview and personal belief system, that is called 'internalization.' One of the ways that internalized inferiority manifests is the belief that you must do something in order to deserve the things you truly want. It is this belief that is the engine of diet culture."

I explained that it took me a long time to understand what internalized inferiority was and how it manifested. It is very difficult to unlearn ideologies that rely upon inferiority (like dieting) without first recognizing that you have feelings of inferiority. The takeaway from that day at the high school was this: the truth is sometimes hidden from us.

When I was learning how to be a good researcher, I was taught the importance of how questions are worded. Sometimes asking someone the most obvious or explicit question isn't the best way to arrive at an actual belief.

So what does inferiority feel like?

When I was new to activism I was convinced that if I had unresolved feelings of inferiority that I would absolutely, without a doubt, know about it. I thought it would be obvious, like the symptoms of a cold or the scrunched-up way my stomach feels when I see someone I really hate while I'm out trying to just get a chili dog and enjoy my life.

It turns out that it's not that simple.

When I was a senior in college I decided I wanted to produce a series of monologues by women of color. I assembled a cast and coached us through writing and production. Each person was encouraged to write a monologue on whatever topic they wanted. I chose to write about my relationship to my breasts, specifically my nipples. I have brown nipples, and for the longest time I had a lot of shame about that fact. I remember once I ended up fooling around with this train conductor in an empty car on the last train back to my apartment. When I took out my breasts he proclaimed with ebullient adoration, "My god, your nipples are so dark!" When he said that, I felt a deep, inexplicable burn in my cheeks.

I realize now that I had internalized the idea that pink nipples were normal and beautiful, and my brown nipples were not. At the time, I didn't understand that this was a manifestation of internalized racism and the education I received in white superiority. I just thought it was a quirk or an individual issue I had.

I remember when I was writing the script for my monologue, some part of me understood that this was a deeper cultural problem and I was evidence of it, but I couldn't let myself see it. I couldn't admit it. I thought that I was too smart and in control for mass media or cultural influences to fool me. I believed that the shame I felt was happening in a vacuum, when in fact it wasn't. It was not an accident that I had anxiety about the parts of my body that marked me as a person of color. I had been taught from an early age that white features were more attractive than dark features. It was just harder to see because no one had flat-out said to me, "You are inferior because you are not white." Rather, the education was subtler, more prolonged, and more obscured. The education in my inferiority wasn't in one place, it was everywhere. Paradoxically, that made it harder to see.

Many times our sense of inferiority is hidden from us. The manifestations of our inferiority ideology might even be experienced as pleasurable. Like the excited feeling you get when someone says that it looks like you've lost weight. Or the pride you feel when you stopped yourself from eating something with sugar in it. Or the elation you may feel when someone you were attracted to finally notices you because you've undertaken steps to make your body more socially acceptable.

Many women do not believe that sexism really, actually exists anymore. And this means they cannot imagine that sexism affects them. I completely understand why. I myself was once someone who didn't see the value of feminism because I didn't understand what misogyny looked like and I couldn't see how it affected my life. I didn't know *how* to look for the signs of misogyny in myself and in the world around me. The signs lived in gestures and feelings, like the way I thought that expressing anger was "unattractive" or the way I was much more patient with men's mistakes than women's. But I couldn't point to any one single person or any one single incident and say, "That's it. That's what's hurting me."

A lot of this has to do with the fact that language and meaning have become increasingly detached. Sexism has become a deeply coded set of behaviors that are difficult to unlock if you don't know how to see them. It can take special access to education and language in order to unveil sexist behavior. Often, that critical language is cast as suspect, overly intellectual, or a product of paranoid fantasy.

We are at a point culturally where it requires more resources than ever to recognize oppression. You must have access to more knowledge and a more nuanced understanding of language to be able to spot its new incarnations. And because the knowledge is more specialized and not obvious to everyone, the person who points out oppression risks being cast as a "professional victim." Women have been told over and over that sexism is a thing of the past: "Stop being a party pooper already!" So being able to identify and call out sexism comes at a high price socially and sometimes professionally.

It's important to recognize that there have been legal advances won by feminists. Women have more rights and access than previous generations could have dreamed of, and certain overt sexist behavior has become taboo. Women now legally have the right to a harassment-free environment at work. This is a wonderful thing, but misogynists have taken advantage of and manipulated the space that has been left in the wake of more obvious manifestations of oppression.

It's excellent that we are protected from overt gender discrimination, but since sexism hasn't been eradicated (it's only been litigated), now women bear the burden of proving that sexism is happening. Many women refuse to speak up because they have a legitimate fear of being ostracized.

It's important to realize that overt sexist behavior is only possible through an entrenched belief in women's inferiority. One of the challenges for feminists is that we as a culture can legislate the overt behavior and yet the ideology can remain intact. This is not a failure on our part but rather the dogged commitment that misogynists have to our dehumanization. Ideologies of oppression are more slippery than rights. They are difficult—if not impossible—to legislate. I think about the hundred small ways that I and other women find ourselves subject to this new "silent" sexism every day.

I think about how the service at the dude-heavy coffee shop down the street from my apartment is friendlier and warmer when I have cleavage exposed (I have run tests!). This reminds me that sexual desirability is always expected of me. Performing feminin-ity extra-special hard feels like a particular expectation of me because I am a fat woman and my bigness always makes others call my gender into question.

I think about the way that it's overwhelm-ingly men who tweet death wishes and harass me online and dox other vocal feminists.

I have to fight the impulse to communi-cate submission when I need something pro-fessionally from a straight man. I know that flirtation is expected by many men when it comes to professional opportunities, and so I sometimes find myself offering a feigned sex-ual interest in them so that they are assuaged and safe in the knowledge that they have con-trol over me even as I am asking for things that will give me more financial freedom.

I think about how much I hate dating because of how exhausting it is dealing with men's pathological desire to wrench power away from me. It starts with the verbiage of my profile. I have to decide between being honest ("I'm a fat feminist") and getting no responses, and using saccharine buzzwords that advertise sexual allure and describe my physical and intellectual qualities as consumable goods that will improve his life ("I'm an articulate, busty BBW"). Once we are seeing each other in real life, then there's a new minefield to navigate. If I just want sex, then he wants more. If I don't want just sex, then I'm needy. I've found that it doesn't matter what I want because most men just want the opposite of what I desire. This is about control.

From the amount of space that male undergraduates take up to the manspreading I witness during my commute, my fat body is frequently attacked on the grounds that I am not beautiful enough to exist because *apparently* that is my job as a woman. I think about the condescending comments I get from men online who tell me that they honestly think I'd be so beautiful if I lost weight—as if that were the goal of my life or my politics. I think about the thousand ways that the women in

my family were silently (and sometimes out-
right) expected to give up their lives, their
dreams, and their desires, so that they could
become the glorified babysitters for the men
in their lives who wanted a legacy but none of
the responsibility of child-rearing. I think of
the way that women are expected to become
mothers, giving up their lives while still being
the object of scorn and pity, while men are
praised for having dad bods.

Men feel the right to control what women
eat—even women they don't know. Emma
Gray wrote an article in 2014 for the *Huffington Post* about a male stranger yelling at
her as she left a frozen-yogurt shop in New
York: "Hey, girl, you shouldn't be eating
that. You're gonna get fat."[1] She conceptualized the comment as both a manifestation of
men's perceived right to control and intimi-
date women in public and this stranger's perceived right to control what she might look
like in the future.

The more we trust our instincts and our
experiences the easier it is to identify sexism. The challenge, of course, is that women
are systematically taught not to trust our
instincts or our experiences. One of the first

times I remember being advised to question myself was during childhood, when I was told that I wasn't hungry even though I was. I was taught as a child that I couldn't trust my body because my mind was playing tricks on me. I was told that I should question my body's demands for food and instead ask myself whether I'm not just actually bored or tired. This was one of my first lessons in self-doubt.

Being pushed into situations where we doubt our experience of reality is called gaslighting. Gaslighting shows up in diet culture a lot. There are real cultural problems—like sexism, body shame, fatphobia, and myriad injustices many of us are dealing with all of the time— and yet we are told over and over again by mainstream narratives that these problems reside within us.

The real problem is that women are angry, and we are trained to turn that anger inward and experience it as shame. And yet we are told—and we believe—that the problem is our body.

The real problem is diet culture, and yet we are told—and we believe—that the problem is our inability to be thin.

The real problem is that we live in a country that promotes size-based bigotry, and yet we are told—and we believe—that the problem is that we are not healthy enough.

The real problem is a culture that uses weight as a proxy for humanity and morality, and yet we are told—and we believe—that the problem is that we don't know how to eat correctly.

The real problem is that women don't feel like we can eat what we want or wear what we want or live how we want, and yet we are told—and we believe—that we can fix this existential crisis through controlling portion size.

The real problem is that our culture is maintained through a vitriolic matrix of sexism, racism, misogyny, transphobia, ableism, healthism, and classism that erodes the physical, spiritual, and mental health of *all* people; and yet we are told—and we believe— that the problem is that we aren't trying hard enough.

Diet culture teaches women that we need to lose weight by any means necessary, thereby reducing us to mere bodies who either do or do not conform to externally set standards. This is dehumanization, plain and simple.

To put it plainly, dieting is a little bit like someone pissing on your leg and then telling you it's raining. Except it's more like someone shitting on your face and then asking you for a dollar and then going into your house and systematically shitting on everything of value that you own and then setting that shit-filled home—that was once filled with the sound of laughter and love but that now's just filled with shit—on fire and then blaming you for it.

Dieting is the outcome of the belief that we don't deserve to live life on our own goddamn terms. And that belief is so entrenched and all-encompassing that it affects even each spoonful of food we eat.

Bros ❤ Thinness: Heteromasculinity and Whiteness

When I was still weight cycling, being thin represented a lot of things to me, but it especially represented access to straight men and heteronormativity, which I thought of as "love." That desire came at a great price. I saw my body as the only commodity I had to trade for love. I did so many destructive things to my body because I think I truly wanted to destroy it—to destroy me. I exercised to the point of exhaustion. I refused to eat the things I loved. I was so anxious about gaining weight and eating that I made myself nauseous all the time. I was nauseous for almost ten years straight. I was in years-long relationships with men who didn't care that I was unhappy and malnourished.

I remember being eighteen years old, on a date with a thirty-eight-year-old secretly married salesman named Cameron. We

had met on a phone personals service. He
bore some resemblance to Mel Gibson circa
Braveheart. Or maybe he just said that often
enough about himself that I believed him.

We were sitting at a booth in a steak
house. He had ordered himself a rib eye and
was enthusiastically chowing down. I remember
trying so hard to be beautiful. I worked at
Mervyn's that summer, and I used my pay-
check and my employee discount to buy new
clothes for our dates. That night I was wearing
uncomfortably tight, white cargo pants and a
green shirt that I'd gotten in the teen section.
It said "double mint" over my breasts. He told
me he liked when I dressed "like a teenager,"
and I wanted to please him. He liked to drive
me around San Francisco and tell me about
all the restaurants where the manager or the
owner or the maître d' knew him. I was from
a small, insulated suburb and was genuinely
impressed by his name-dropping. I had made
a habit of trying to be unobtrusive by ordering
a small plate or simply eating from my date's
plate. I think that night I might have been
feeling particularly excited because we were
at a fancy restaurant in the Financial Dis-
trict. I wanted to order my own plate rather

than sit there watching him. I told him I wanted to order something. He stopped, knife and fork in hand, and sighed. "You're not going to eat it anyway," he said in a matter-of-fact tone verging on exasperation. And went back to eating.

I felt so ashamed. It felt like there was a silent expectation that I would do whatever I had to do to remain my size—but preferably smaller. I was working so hard, and the meal (whether I was going to eat it or not) symbolized his recognition of this work. The meal represented the fulfillment of the reciprocal understanding of our respective gender roles: I had done my job as a woman not to eat, and I expected him to play his role and buy me a gift. I was further embarrassed because if he'd noticed that I never ate, then I was failing at hiding my dieting; the mask had slipped and he had known all along that I was trying too hard to be pretty. My dieting was an act of service, but it was understood that I could never make it seem like work. Like the way a waitress must never seem like she isn't having a great time.

For me, hetero romance was as much of a fantastical story as dieting was. I wanted my life to follow particular plot points, and I thought that my weight was how I could control the narrative.

Romance aside, it's important to recognize that misogyny and men play a major role in the maintenance of fatphobia.

Rather than recognizing the multiplicity of feminine expression and feminine power (regardless of sex assignment at birth, ability, size, the presence or absence of modesty or money), women in pursuit of thinness become complicit in their own dehumanization and therefore become agents of misogyny.

A few years ago I was having dinner with one of my closest friends and a bunch of her friends. We sat at the big table in her dining room passing plates of roasted root vegetables covered in goat cheese, pouring red wine, and covering a polite range of topics. I will tell you right now that I hate dinner parties with respectable people. I like dinner parties with my friends, who frequently talk about anal sex and the last time someone had the nerve to be utterly basic in public. This particular group kept dinner conversation focused on safe topics: weather, recent travel, tasteful boasts of career success, and impending rituals like weddings, babies, or home ownership. I listened on with a mildly derisive anthropological interest.

After dessert, people started to leave until there were just three of us left: me, my close friend, and another woman. The third woman was stylish, smart, striking, and charming. She was funny and had amazingly shiny hair. Jokes quickly turned into "real talk" once we got a little drunker. She admitted to us that she was thinking of dropping out of her PhD program at an elite institution. She seemed really upset, really torn up about it. She loved her program, she told us.

We asked her why in the world she would give up something she cared so much about. She told us that she really wanted a relationship and a family with a man, and that she had always had trouble because she was almost six feet tall. Now that she was nearing thirty, she was starting to panic. She had tried to date, but found that the combination of her height and her level of education acted as a "double whammy." She'd been on dates where men flat-out told her that she was too much. She reflected to us sadly that although she couldn't change her height, she could change whether or not she had a PhD.

It still makes me cry every time I think of her. I suspect that her story is not unique. Women strategically debase ourselves consistently because of desires for romance, especially in straight relationships. I think what made that evening unique was her willingness to talk about it.

I asked her not to leave her program. I told her how much compassion I felt for her. I shared that I understood her story better than she could probably even imagine. We were both big women—in different ways— who were trying to find meaningful connections with straight dudes in a deeply broken culture. I never saw her again, and I have no idea whether she left her program or not. I sometimes regret that I didn't vehemently tell her that she was wrong about men. But I didn't because I knew she wasn't.

We are taught that men are the key to happiness and fulfillment. We fear that without heterosexual marriage and childbearing we cannot become people who matter or "real" adults. It is this nexus of desire and fear that is the breeding ground for self-destructive behavior like dieting. Rather than being taught that you deserve love simply because you are a person, you are taught that love is something people must earn through particular socially sanctioned methods. For many women, that method is weight control.

It's important to recognize that men become both the stand-ins for cultural approval and the enforcers of normativity, even though they themselves are also subject to the realities of our oppressive gender paradigm. It is often at their hands that women and girls learn that their emotional, professional, and romantic well-being depends on proximity to men.

Misogyny manifests differently depending on how your body is positioned in the sexist schema. Let me be clear: all women are subjugated. Thin women get dehumanized just as fat women do, but it often looks different. Very thin women are positioned in far more public positions (as wives and girlfriends), while fat women are positioned in far more private positions (as lovers and secrets).

Even among fat-bodied women, there are variations in treatment based on behavior and social status. A fat woman who is cisgender is likely to be treated differently than a fat woman who is trans. Because both fat women and trans women are acutely marginalized, relationships with fat or trans women are often hidden from the public. Fat trans women experience the violence that exists at the nexus of sexism, fatphobia, and transphobia. Race is another mitigating factor. The lighter you are the more culturally valued you are. So, whiteness or light skin can soften fat-negative bias, whereas dark-skinned women may experience increased hostility due to the combined effects of colorism and fatphobia.

Fat women who are willing to accept their cultural position as inferior get treated differently than fat women who are politicized. For example, I have been fat my entire life, but my fatness was less a source of anxiety before I was a fat feminist. Before I was a fat feminist, I was willing to do more work to "compensate" for my lower social standing. I performed more sexual labor. I did not set boundaries. I apologized frequently for my weight and accepted blame when my partners and others criticized my body. Once I knew how to advocate for myself and set limits, dating became significantly more challenging—

even though I was a fat woman both before my introduction to feminism and after.

What we must realize is that it's not thinness that is being eroticized. What is being eroticized is the submission thinness represents in our culture. Thinness is a secondary characteristic. The true commodity is the willingness of women to acquiesce to cultural control.

Controlling women's body size is about controlling women's lives. This claim to control is based on fantasies of masculine superiority bolstered by the culture. This control does not just apply to thinness.

Fatness and thinness mean different things in different places. Right now as you're reading this book there are places in our world where women are being ritualistically fattened in order to become more romantically competitive. In parts of Mauritania and Niger, fat rolls and stretch marks are considered the height of feminine beauty.

Just as women in the West undertake uncomfortable and sometimes-harmful methods to become ever thinner, these women are at times force-fed or consume dangerous weight-gaining medications designed for animals in order to fit a radically different, though equally damaging, beauty ideal. I read about European and American anthropologists in Mauritania who couldn't believe the first time they witnessed women in these areas getting weighed at the clinic. They put more clothes on before getting on the scale, so they would be heavier, rather than removing clothes the way women almost reflexively do in the West.

The years I spent being taught fatphobia by my peers growing up, and then by media, destroyed my sense of self. By the time the boys at school were through teaching me that my greatest accomplishment in life would be to lose enough weight to date one of them, I had no idea what I actually needed or wanted. All that was left in the wake of my dazzling and silly personality was a desire to never feel like an outsider again. Being weird and bossy and theatrical and curious had always been the best things about me. But those qualities attracted attention, and attention was emotionally dangerous. All that was left was a traumatized approval-seeking girl with no sense of her own magic. It was disproportionately at the hands of boys my age that I was taught that I was worthless. The justification was that they didn't find me desirable and this was a punishable offense to them.

Paradoxically I didn't fight back because I thought their behavior was my fault.

I was convinced that I could control their behavior and make it all better if I just tried harder to become their idea of beautiful. What they were attempting to teach me were the lessons that many girls and women before me have been taught:

- Men and boys are allowed to teach women and girls about compliance with social expectations of desirability without our consent.
- Men and boys are allowed to use systems of sexual and emotional approval and disapproval to confirm masculine superiority and ideologies of control—offering sexual and romantic attention to women and girls whose bodies conform to social standards of beauty while socially isolating or punishing those whose bodies do not. Both behaviors are based on dehumanization.

These behaviors create an intense sense of dependency on masculine approval, which is gauged exclusively through sexual and romantic interest. This leads to the low self-worth that facilitates things like disordered eating and rape culture.

Misogyny works in tandem with white supremacy to build a population of women that is pliant and easily manipulated in order to carry out the oppressive needs of the culture and the state as they currently exist.

It's important to recognize that the desire to be thin is actually part of a drive to be compliant with current Western expectations of feminine submission and second-class citizenship. This model of feminine submission is deeply informed by whiteness. As Patricia Hill Collins, Audre Lorde, and bell hooks have all pointed out, white femininity has historically played a colluding role in the maintenance of white supremacy and hetero-patriarchy, acting as a sort of wedge or intermediary third party that solidifies the power brokered between white men of influence and everyone else. This agreement has cost white women full citizenship, but it is through the promise of second-class citizenship that they are invested in maintaining the current gender/race paradigm.

I want to end this section with a sobering observation. When I work with women who want to stop dieting, we will often make a lot of emotional progress until we get to romance. The women who envision spending their lives with men or who are partnered with a fat-negative person are much more likely to return to dieting. The women who either have a fat-positive partner or who are queer are less likely. This is not to say that there are no straight women with incredible fat-positive partners, or that there are no queers who experience fatphobia in their relationships. This observation is anecdotal, but it's telling.

No single feminist can fix the legacy of misogyny that continues to cycle through and destroy our lives. What I can tell you is that you are not alone in your stultifying disappointment or (occasional? constant?) sense of hopelessness, and that you don't have to acquiesce to the sexist forces that seek to make you small—both metaphorically and literally.

Fatphobia Is the New Language of Classism and Racism

There is no shortage of examples when it comes to the ways that fat people create cultural anxiety. It is no accident that fat people are underrepresented in the workplace, academia, and mass media. When we *are* visible, we are portrayed as unintelligent, lacking in grace or complexity, inherently amusing, abject, and either sexually insatiable or lacking any sexual desire. Fat people are largely absent from meaningful portrayals of the future, similar to disabled people, trans people, and people of color.

Body size has some really compelling connections to cultural anxiety about class, race, and gender. Discussions of and feelings about class and race and gender have been transposed onto discussions of and feelings about fat people. I want to talk about the connections between fatphobia and class, race, and gender using the example of a campaign that was launched in January 2012 in Georgia.

Children's Healthcare of Atlanta launched a scare tactic campaign targeting "childhood obesity" called Strong4Life. They purchased ad space on billboards and television. The ads featured stark images of unsmiling children in gray scale with bold red lettering that read WARNING in all caps across their bellies. There was swift backlash against the campaign, but the verbiage splayed across these kids' bodies created a window into some of the less-often articulated anxieties about fat people and the ways that obesity rhetoric becomes a stand-in for other cultural anxieties.

These ads did the very thing to fat people that the culture does all the time. These children are dehumanized by the desire to use their bodies to tell a story about a culturally perceived problem. Their complexity is flattened and rendered invisible through the monochromatic story. Further, their unhappy expressions render them a cautionary tale. They are actually being warned against as if their fatness were contagious. This style of alarmist advertising subtly evokes the anxiety that fat is communicable through proximity to fat bodies. This illogical fear of infection is, in part, why fat people are socially ostracized.

What I found most interesting about these ads was the story that each of them told about class, race, and gender. I am absolutely positive that the person who came up with the copy for each of these had no intention of unveiling such a complex and nuanced set of cultural anxieties, yet it is this inadvertence that makes it so powerful. The truth comes through if you know how to see it, and it bums me out to no end that it took years of study- ing nearly inscrutable high theory to be able to decipher truth from a bunch of muddled, indirect language.

There were four ads in total. I will describe and analyze three of them.

The first image is of a fat prepubescent white boy around ten years old. He is wear- ing a dark, tight, unbuttoned polo shirt and dark jeans. His hands are in his pockets, his shoulders pulled back. Across his belly there is a line of text that reads: "Fat prevention begins at home and the buffet line," which speaks indirectly to poor and working-class people, and to mothers specifically. You will not find a lot of upper-middle-class people at buffets because they defy the affluent and middle-class value of restraint. The idea of restraint suggests that "less is more," and that eating as much as you want is a sign of immorality and the lack of discipline that characterizes the undeserving poor. Restraint is a concept poor people often can't afford to adopt because the maxim "less is more" is not literal. Restraint is only fun or laudable when the threat of actual loss or insufficiency is nowhere on the horizon. When you're broke, "less" is a very negative and often terrifying thing. "Less" is not a choice; it is a physical reality that has material and emotional consequences.

The clientele of buffets is largely comprised of working-class and poor people who are successfully maximizing budgets by getting as much value as they can for the least money. This economic decision is intuitive, and in fact it is the concept of restraint that is contrived. By calling out the buffet line the creators of the ad are perpetuating class-based bigotry while also creating deniability by not explicitly naming poor and working-class people.

Further, this ad is speaking specifically—

though not explicitly—to women because we know statistically that women are still the disproportionate meal preparers and providers for children. Some of this disproportionate parenting comes from the reality that women earn less money and, for a straight couple, it makes more economic sense for the lower-earning parent to stay at home. Perhaps this is because feeding children is still perceived as female-gendered labor, as it is part of caretaking. Regardless of the reason for this disproportionate parenting, the ad again avoids an overt reference to mothers, but because of the reality of sexism, they are clearly the intended audience.

This "buffet" reference speaks to working-class women without actually saying "Dear poor women, stop feeding your children in a way that feels intuitive to you. Your parenting is toxic to your children."

The second ad depicts a fat prepubescent white girl, also around ten. She has long, light brown hair and is wearing a long-sleeved striped T-shirt with jeans. Her frowning expression stands in marked contrast to the way white girls are usually portrayed in popular media. Her arms are crossed over her chest, her shoulders hunched slightly. The phrase "It's hard to be a little girl if you're not" is splayed across her belly, telling a story about gender anxiety, (inadvertently) questioning whether a fat girl is even a girl at all. The gender anxiety at the root of this idea is very familiar to me because I grew up feeling like I was straddling masculinity and femininity. I grew up being told I was a girl, and yet because of my size, the behavior I experienced from my peers felt more in line with masculinity. At home I would watch movies that showed me that girls get treated like dainty, delicate flowers and boys get treated roughly. At school, I was treated like a big tough boy, not like a flower. So, for example, during play time with other girls, we would often enact scenes from *The Baby-Sitters Club* or other books and shows we loved. When it came time to play out the romantic parts, I always played the boy, without question. We never even discussed it because it was just silently understood that boys are bigger than girls, and I was bigger than everyone, and therefore I was the obvious choice to play the boy.

I remember for the entirety of fourth grade,

every day at lunch my best friend Lorna and I would reenact the romance between *BSC*'s Mary Anne Spier and Logan Bruno. They were the only long-standing couple in the book series, and everyone I knew desperately wanted to be Mary Anne. I desperately wanted to be Mary Anne, not just because I was a supremely horny and suppressed Christian, but also because I wanted evidence that I was desirable.

Lorna was a nerdy Chinese girl who wore glasses, and I was a nerdy Mexican girl who wore glasses. Our most significant difference was that I was big and she was small. I wanted to be Mary Anne SO BADLY, but I never once even suggested that we switch roles. I was too afraid for the unspoken truth to be out in the open. I felt the looming rejection, and I was scared of what would happen if we actually said the words. So I played a boy every day. I would pick her up. I would make her feel small and beautiful. I would put on a Southern twang just like Logan had. I would suck up my desire and my most vulnerable wishes so that the story could be believable.

So when I saw this ad for the first time, it hit me. It resonated. It *is* hard to be a little girl, if you're not. Fatness disrupts the cultural obsession with sexual differentiation, the gender binary, and the idea that women need to be clearly and visibly distinguishable from men. Fat women have bigger bodies, and often more strength because of those bigger bodies. Fat men may have bigger chests and softer bodies.

The cultural treatment of fat men's bodies centers heavily on sexist rhetoric. Fat men are often cast as feminine. I've noted that many instances of fatphobia directed at men (though certainly not all) are about the anxiety that fat men will be perceived as womanlike. So I believe that it is the deep cultural hatred of the feminine that leads to *some* of the instances of fatphobia that men experience.

While researching this phenomenon for an article, I noticed three themes pointing to sexist anxiety about fat men's bodies. First, there was anxiety about chemical feminization, the concern that fatness increases the conversion of testosterone into estrogen. In a *Salon* article entitled "Sex Researchers: 'Size' Does Matter" (subtitle: "Study shows that fatter men last longer in bed. Should Americans rejoice?"), Judy Mandelbaum writes, "Men with excess fat showed higher levels of the female estradiol sex hormone. This substance apparently disrupted their bodies' natural 'male' neurotransmitter chemicals and slowed their progression towards orgasm. Ironically, *the less masculine their bodies appeared*, the better lovers they proved to be."[1] No other possible conclusions or analyses of this finding are discussed

Second, there was anxiety about fatness obstructing the visibility of men's genitals. A popular meme was what I started calling the "fat castration" meme: the idea that fat men cannot find their penis or are otherwise figuratively castrated by their fat.

Finally, I found anxiety expressed toward fat men developing breasts. In a *Men's Health* article on "banishing your man boobs," the author writes, "You probably love a great set of breasts—as long as you're not the one sporting them."[2] The language draws parallels between compulsory heterosexuality, masculinity, and body size in one fell swoop— subtly policing the boundaries of sexuality by pointing out that only women should have breasts and that men should be attracted to them. If you have "man boobs," then you are blurring the culturally sanctioned bifurcation between men and women. Further, since fatness is rendered as an individual choice in popular cultural discourse, it is taboo for a man to opt into a more feminine gender presentation since femininity is debased through misogyny.

So when I see this Strong4Life ad, I see some of the same projection of anxiety about gender onto this girl's body. I also see the role of white femininity in the construction of gender, and the way that the chubby white girl in the ad creates tension between ideal femininity and fat embodiment.

The tone of the verbiage shifts in the third ad, which depicts a fat Black girl. She is maybe eleven or twelve and looks like she has just begun puberty. She is wearing a white baby tee and jeans. Her black hair is shoulder length and pulled back in a white headband. Her hands are in her pockets, her shoulders hunched forward a little. Her lips are pursed, positioning her femininity as different from the white girl's. The language becomes more personal in her ad, and the scope of the message smaller: "Fat may be funny to you but it's killing me." The only ad of the three that makes reference to the individual unit, the self. The subtle shift in language—from passive voice to second person—felt significant, but I didn't quite have the language to articulate why. I asked my friend Sirius Bonner, a diversity and equity consultant, fat woman, and Black feminist who lives in Portland, Oregon, to share her thoughts on this image. She told me, "Fat Black women have a very particular spot in the public consciousness. They are considered inherently humorous. The use of the word 'funny' is an othering reference to that 'inherent humor' that Black women are considered to possess. The shift from passive voice to second person takes the conversation out of the realm of the universal, reminding the viewer of the Black/white binary." She pointed out that white bodies can be discussed as stand-ins for all people, but Black bodies are not allowed that same versatility in our culture.

I looked back at the image after talking to Sirius and saw that the girl's fatness had become a vehicle to leverage a critique against Black people. The verbiage rendered the treatment of her fat body as something that implicated her community. Through the "you" reference, the viewer is called to participate in the racist act of blaming and pathologizing Black people in the name of public health.

The idea behind the ads is that being fat is a life-threatening affliction and that fat people should be avoided because we are vectors of disease and death. Right now, our culture equates fatness with mortality and ill-health, but in order to understand this issue from a social justice perspective we must widen the frame and allow complexity to enter our field of vision. When I look at the literature on the subject, I find glaring holes in the deduction process.

There is compelling evidence that racism kills people. There is compelling evidence that living with the stress of poverty leads to a number of mental health challenges. There is compelling evidence that weight-based discrimination leads to heightened levels of stress and anxiety that suppress the function of major organs. And, there is evidence that fatphobia leads to shortened life expectancy.[3] But racism, poverty, and weight-based bigotry are all social problems. It is through victim-blaming narratives that we cast these social issues as individual ones that can be solved through bootstrapping and consumerism. Unfortunately, these "solutions" are only survival mechanisms, at best. As we undertake them, we only dig ourselves further into the very oppression we are attempting to escape.

What Early Fat Activism Taught Me

In 2010 I was introduced to fat activism while I was getting my master's degree in sexuality studies. I had been interviewing fat women about how their size had affected the development of their gender. At the time, the world of fat activism was small; news traveled fast, introductions were eagerly made, and there was an almost electric feeling to all of it.

Even though fat feminism has roots in 1960s Jewish lesbian politics, this iteration of the fat movement was, in many ways, a campy and irreverent offshoot that was just beginning to gain traction. Everyone on the planet who was doing anything visible around fat politics knew everyone else. There were small pockets in the Bay Area, the Midwest, the Pacific Northwest, New York, Canada, the UK, and Australia. I would later meet fat activists in Mexico, Chile, Italy, Austria,

and New Zealand. Through the fat grape-
vine, someone had found out that I was doing
research on fatness and all of a sudden I was
meeting fat activists. They introduced me to
people they knew. They recommended books.
The most memorable and impactful introduction came when someone asked me, "Have
you heard of the NOLOSE conference?" I said
no and asked her what it was. She said it was
a conference for fat queers and that I had to
go. So a few weeks later I found myself taking
a train and then a bus to a hotel in Oakland.

I had no idea how significant stepping off
that bus was going to be. I was a new kid in
a new town—a mildly frumpy wallflower who
was about to have her goddamn mind blown.
I dragged my sad, navy-blue suitcase down
the concrete, through the decorative rock garden, and onto the hotel property, pushing my
glasses up the bridge of my nose all the while.

As I was making my way through the
breezeway, I heard the sound of splashing
and women's laughter. I could smell the chlo-
rine from the pool. And then I saw them:
a group of fat babes. I had never seen fat
women in a group like this. I had never seen
fat women in cute bathing suits. I had never

seen fat women in cute bathing suits lounging and floating and chatting in public, at a pool no less. There were fatties floating in the water, lounging in chairs getting a tan, complimenting other fatties about how good they looked, and reading poolside. I was frozen in place by the sight of them—unapologetically, blissfully living. I had never seen women like them—women like us—living without any discernable trace of shame. They were doing what I believed fat people could never do.

And then from stage left came this high-femme redhead. She was wearing a red vintage bathing suit with white polka dots and a huge pair of cat-eye sunglasses. Her large breasts, belly, and thighs were hardly contained. And trailing behind her was a boy holding a parasol over her so she wouldn't burn. She had the glamour of a movie star, and a body that wasn't so different from my own.

And in that moment I was converted. I gave myself over to the Ultra Mega Badass Fat Babe Lifestyle when I saw her. In her, I saw the possibility of an entirely different life. It was like those transformation teen movies, but rather than my body changing, something else happened. I realized after years of dieting that I had been trying to change the wrong thing. I didn't need to change my body; I needed to change the way I felt about it.

When I was introduced to fat activism, it was a uniquely and resoundingly queer political movement. Fat people, and the needs of fat people, were at the center of the politic. The movement had an anti-assimilationist framework that I found both familiar and wonderfully provocative. We ruthlessly questioned notions like "health" and "fitness," and talked about the ways that fat people were threatening because we interrupted heteronormative time lines (though not often using that exact verbiage).[1]

Liberation was central to the conversations I was witnessing and participating in. There was a recognition that "acceptance" was not a desired outcome because absorption into the racist, patriarchal, and fatphobic culture that has systematically dehumanized you isn't exactly a "win." Acceptance is kind of like marrying that dude in high school who called you a fat pig every day for four years and then ran into you eight years later when you looked a lot cuter (because when you weren't living under the reign of his emotional violence you actually had space to put together outfits you loved and get an amazing haircut) and then asks you to date him and you say yes because you are so traumatized that you can only experience his violence as love. Right?

As fat activism began to be eclipsed by body positivity,[2] there was a shift away from a liberation framework in favor of assimilation. I think I can say as lovingly as possible that body positivity has gained and will continue to gain traction with its newfound focus. As a straight, cisgender woman, I honestly understand the deep and hypnotic draw of assimilation. The closer you perceive your access to ideal citizenship to be, the harder it is to want something bigger, better. But fat activism taught me that being accepted by the very people who made me feel less than human isn't enough. So why settle?

Over the years, I began to find myself in more and more body positive spaces and fewer fat activism spaces. My drift toward body positive spaces felt unintentional, but I know it was facilitated by a number of things: my straightness, my access to higher education and ability to code-switch into white spaces, my access to and interest in publishing, my sunshiny disposition, my desire and ability to monetize my work, and my size and shape relative to other fat people. I feel a lot of ambivalence about all of this, but the point of the story is that this transition was, honestly, startling in a number of key ways.

First, within the body positivity movement, the demands were much more difficult to decipher. I was pretty sure that liberation was not a demand, but I wasn't sure what was. Equality? Cute dates? I quickly discovered that it was no accident that I had no idea what the demands were. It was through silence that this body positive movement spoke most clearly and loudly to mainstream culture. The rules of femininity state that it is not "ladylike" to make demands or set boundaries. In many ways, that is why feminists are often masculinized and consequently demonized. So the women-led body positivity movement's choice to make no clear demands is about the willingness to sacrifice rights and freedom for the maintenance of an oppressive construct. Trying to decipher the silence reminded me of the lessons my grandma used to give me about dealing with men. Silence was a very powerful tool. Silence, according to my grand-mother, was the appropriate response to verbal abuse or sexual dissatisfaction, even coercion. Silence was the antidote to a fight. You got a man to pay for your meal, not by asking, but by *not* asking. I learned to excuse myself at the end of a date so we wouldn't be left with the untidy conversation around pay-ment and the power dynamics that live at the core of that conversation.

Silence is a very gendered and highly racialized tactic.

It was the silence in the body positivity movement that allowed traction to be gained. If there's nothing clearly articulated then there's nothing to violate, no need to call any-one out if there's nothing to call out.

Second, there was less a desire for freedom than for absorption. I began to notice that there was a real preoccupation with prescrip-tive gender behavior. After years of being around women who pushed back against the oppressive Susie Sunshine archetype, I was starting to feel a real sense that these women didn't want to be impolite, didn't want to raise their voices, and wanted to make politi-cal strides through hugs and genteel working lunches. It was white femininity if I ever saw it. And even though it was never said out loud, their behavior indicated a commitment to the status quo that was staggering to me, especially after having spent nearly a decade in queer feminist spaces.

An incredible amount of energy was spent trying to make sure that everyone was nice and nonthreatening. Conversations about accountability were quickly discarded as petty manifestations of rudeness. Discussions about history and political ideology were cast as terrifyingly intellectual. And for the first time, there were women who were vociferously defending diets and weight loss. Because they eschewed hard conversations, it was impossible to be real with them. It's important to be clear that this performance of white femininity and white gentility is just that—a performance. As starched and polished and pearl-bedecked as that performance is, at its core is the notion of submission and the idea that through submission we can maintain privilege.

Third, the movement's vision felt much, much smaller. As I went from organizing primarily with queer people to organizing primarily with straight cis women, I was shocked to find that the scope of vision shifted drastically from a clearly articulated desire for human rights to an implied desire to primarily access privilege. The queers I had met in fat activism were proudly politicized, having spent years and sometimes decades learning about oppression and being unabashed in their pursuit of justice. The straight women I began to meet were more politically demure. They were preoccupied with the avoidance of being considered mean and had a strong distaste for other women they perceived as "hostile" in their political stances. They wanted a movement that was nice and supportive, not emotionally nuanced or accountability driven.

They seemed to want, primarily, clothing they liked, more substantive access to heterosexual romance, and the right to claim that they were radical no matter their actual politics. Clothing and romance had always been really important parts of and conversations within fat activism, for sure. But the political demands and expectations didn't begin and end there. I found that in organizing with other straight women, their expectations had a dangerously low ceiling.

Sadly I found that at the core of their indifference toward freedom or liberation was their proximity to men. Some part of them knew that their relationship to men would shift if they could admit the truth—that men played a large role in maintaining their subjugated status. I wish I could say that they were scared that once they admitted the truth and sought accountability that their desire to be close to their current or potential partners would change. But the truth was they were scared that if they spoke the truth that men wouldn't want to be with *them*; they would have become those "difficult" women they had disliked previously. They were still taking care of men; for many, they were taking care of men they hadn't even met yet, men they hoped to meet in the future.

Straightness has long kept women from organizing and from demanding not only what is ours but also what is right and just. It is both our fear and our investment that holds us hostage. I honestly don't know exactly how to reconcile the imagined future spent with a dude by my side and the reality that I know an anti-assimilationist queer politic is the one that inspires the deepest and has the realest resonance for me. But I do know that freedom is the only way. And any movement that does not center collective liberation is not one in which I can invest.

In the Future, I'm Fat

I write very good personal ads. I know that the age of the ad has largely come and gone, but I've always loved the idea that my first interaction with someone was linguistic rather than visual. In the realm of digital romance, language is used in a very pragmatic, outcome-driven way. People tend to focus on statistics, measurements, desires, goals, and hobbies. My ads are less like lists and more like full-length confessional manifestos. All of the distance and suspicion I convey while on dates is counterbalanced by the intimate nature of what I've written before the date.

Men in San Francisco, I've found, tend to be very intrigued by my ads. I've noticed that I've developed a regional voice because when I place the same ads when I'm traveling I often get emails that rhetorically pose questions like, "What is wrong with you?" My ads detail not only where I live and what I like but also my passion for nail polish, jasmine and gardenias, tiramisu and cheesecake, particular scents I find evocative of particular times, the way my face looks in the morning—the fact that I am incapable of actual intimacy but am very invested in the quickly won, shallow intimacy that can only be had between strangers who like the idea of having sex with each other, probably, once.

I had written one such ad in 2014 and attracted a very eager doctor dude. After exchanging a few emails, he asked for "permission" to "aggressively pursue" me. He sounded like a psychopath and so naturally I was interested. I've noticed men in traditional professions are skittish about sharing what exactly they do. So it wasn't until we were at this Peruvian restaurant chewing on tiny, crispy octopus tentacles near the Haight that he divulged that he was an "obesity researcher."

He followed this up quickly with telling me that he was a big fan of my work. The whole thing was very confusing. Thankfully, more than connection, I love a deeply alienating weirdo who has watched YouTube videos I made in my bedroom about how to turn garden accents into hair accessories or how to "sluttify" any outfit with only scissors and the will to release any claim to respectability. I'm not sure exactly what kept me on that date: perhaps it was that I wasn't woke enough to see what he represented, perhaps I liked what he represented, perhaps I was willing to give him a pass for pathologizing people like me because he was fat too.

He had an interesting story. He said he had always identified as an "overeater." He said he liked food a lot and ate frequently, and had always been thin. All of a sudden, at around thirty-five, something kind of unexpected happened. His behavior didn't change, but for reasons he couldn't quite grasp he went from being a thin person to being a fat one.

On the date he asked me, "Wouldn't your life be easier, though, if you were thin?"

The answer to this question is simple: no.

My life wouldn't be easier if I were thin. My life would be easier if this culture wasn't obsessed with oppressing me because I'm fat. The solution to a problem like bigotry is not to do everything in our power to accommodate the bigotry. It is to get rid of the bigotry.

In the dreams I have of my future, I am fat. This simple fact was hard won. For years and years, I could not accept the possibility that I would be fat forever. I had internalized fatphobia so deeply that I believed my life wasn't worth living if I wasn't going to some-day transform into a thin person. I didn't think I deserved to have good things because I was fat. Like many women, I had a ward-robe filled with clothes that didn't fit me. I didn't let anyone take photos of me. I cut up the pictures of me that did end up surfacing. This inability to see yourself in the future is a product of believing there is no room for you in the culture that surrounds you. The future, it turns out, is a lot about the present.

The allure of diet culture is a life lived in the future. The future is a hermetically sealed unreality that possesses none of the limits— or the potential for magic—of the present. The present is messy, sweaty, filled with longing and sometimes anger and sometimes sadness. The present holds your body in all the imperfection that makes it real.

The future represents possibility to many.

My obsession with my thin future was about disembodiment. It was about disassociating completely from myself, the present and my body. In the narrative I created about the future, I was the author of my life. I deeply longed to feel that sense of ownership, but I didn't know how to access it because I had been emotionally battered so severely by a fat-hating, woman-hating culture.

I had felt that I could earn that authorship through compliance. I couldn't bear the reality that I was living in. So I jettisoned my emotional self out of the present and into another time. It was a beautiful time filled with all the things I wanted most, which I felt I didn't deserve because I wasn't in a "good" body. I violently deleted my true self from the story by always focusing on an anesthetized future filled with other people who also knew how to conform successfully. I never thought of those people as good or bad. I thought of them as real, and my fat self as an in-between space I was temporarily occupying. I became complicit with them in the destruction of my past and all that my failure represented: my undisciplined body, my lack of feminine grace, my inability to be white enough, my rage, and my inability to assimilate completely into American culture. I didn't think of it that way back then, but that was the truth of it.

I conceptualized that in my future I would be free because I would be thin, but I was wrong. In that future I imagined, it's not that I was free. Far from it. Any future that doesn't center the eradication of oppression and collective freedom is not a future worth imagining. In that future I imagined I was no longer subject to fatphobia because I was thin, but I didn't realize that it wasn't fatphobia that had gone away. There was no me. The fantasy of and longing for a thin body became a way of making the oppression that was breaking my heart, breaking me, more bearable. It didn't occur to me that there was anything wrong with the idea that anyone—let alone an entire culture—would bully me into believing there was something fundamentally wrong with me and that I needed to change it. It never occurred to me that the standard of normal to which I was subscribing was violent, and always had been. I thought I could *earn* my way out of oppression, but I realize now that nothing is farther from the truth. I had lost sight of my right to freedom and my right to live a life free from oppression. I had lost sight that those things are my born right.

You cannot earn freedom through conformity. You cannot buy your way in. And we can only claim it when we recognize it is already ours.

I Want Freedom

For a very long time I wanted to lose weight more than I wanted absolutely anything else. I believed that life would begin later. I would wear a bikini later. I would be happy later. I would wear short shorts, go on dates, feel beautiful, wear bright-pink lipstick later. I would travel the world, enjoy cupcakes, and smile with complete abandon in pictures later (when my cheeks were smaller and I didn't have a double chin). I would love myself later.

I want to be completely clear with you about what dieting was about for me. It was not just about eating carrots, fat-free pop-corn, low-calorie Pop-Tarts, or fat-free, sugar-free, gluten-free frozen yogurt. It was not just about weighing myself once, twice, or some-times ten times a day. It was not just the pure joy I felt when I'd gone down a pound or the intense shame and self-loathing when

I gained it back. It was not just about the "willpower" and the jumping jacks and the pedometer that tells you how many miles you walked this week. It was not just about skipping dessert or sleeping through dinner. It was not just about food journals or crying in front of the mirror while I squeezed my fat loathingly.

I realize now that all those years I dedicated to losing weight and hating my body were actually about a misguided attempt to be free. Yes, I dieted because I believed that it was only through weight loss that I could deserve to travel, wear cute clothes, and go on lots of dates with people I was hot for. But more than that, I wanted the stuff that those things represented: happiness, love, joy, and, most importantly, freedom. I was trying to starve my way into freedom. I had been taught to believe that weight loss was the key to all my heart's greatest desires, but the truth is that it wasn't. Because you can't find self-love by walking a path paved by self-hatred.

I had been taught that dieting was the path to freedom, and it took me a long time to realize that this was one of the greatest lies ever told. With dieting, everything depended on me accepting that I was the one to blame because I was fat. With dieting, I had to admit that there was nothing wrong or sick about a culture that taught me how to hate myself. With dieting, I had to believe that the trouble and the problem resided within me, not outside of me. I was intoxicated by the notion of this individual power. Even as it was eating me alive, it was feeding me the idea that I could have anything I wanted, that the more I sacrificed the more I gained.

I realize now that all those times I had said, "I want to be thin," I actually meant:

I want to be loved.

I want to be happy.

I want to be seen.

I want to be free.

We are taught that thin is synonymous with beauty, power, and love. But, in fact, it is not. Beauty is not something women earn; it is something people are. Power is not achieved through the dogged pursuit of homogeneity; it is something that is innate within us and that is strengthened by nonconformity. Love is not something people earn through obedience; it is each person's birthright. We cannot starve our way into being loved, into being free.

The truth is that right now women and girls are starving themselves every day. They are going on their first diet before they even turn ten. They are being told to wear things that hide or "flatter" their body. They are food policed and fat shamed by their classmates and coworkers. They are obsessively exercising to the point of pain or injury. They can find no peace until they have sweat out the last calorie they consumed. They are dreaming of taking a knife to their belly. They are getting romantically rejected and ghosted and blaming themselves—believing that if they just lose a little more weight, then someone who's not even worth their time will call them back. They are obsessively looking at food labels. They are avoiding entire sections of the grocery store because they don't think they can control the impulse to binge if they see something delicious. They are religiously avoiding protein and fat. They are stepping onto scales multiple times a day. They are avoiding being photographed or only allowing their lives to be documented if they "look thin." They are unable to imagine themselves in the future at their current size. They are accepting unacceptable relationships and sexual experiences because they feel like they don't deserve any better. They are unable to even access what they want because they have experienced so many years of being told that what their body is telling them is wrong.

This is not a picture of wellness.

This is not a picture of success.

This is not a picture of normalcy.

And yet this is the reality of many, many women's lives. This is what diet culture looks like. This is what my life looked like for nearly two decades.

It's hard to neatly compress twenty years of life. I would be remiss if I didn't include the wild beauty in my own story. I got caught up in a cultural whirlwind so much bigger and uglier than I could have ever dreamed, but I lived a lot during those years that I was trying to survive. Life somehow found a way to burst out of my fear, like flowers through a crack in the sidewalk.

I always thought it was so funny or maybe sad that it was in large part because of fatphobia that I was forced to find alternatives to my small, conservative town. Thanks to fatphobia no one would date me and so I developed a sexual and romantic resiliency like no other. I immediately saw the potential of the internet for outcasts like me, and so I familiarized myself with new technology quicker than my classmates even though my family didn't have a computer in the house. In some ways, I think my early and intimate relationship with cyberspace is why I became a cyberfeminist. I got good at writing and articulating things because I was navigating word-heavy mediums. My first dates should have been at McDonald's or Applebee's, but because I was meeting dudes who had to pay for phone personals services, instead they were at fancy restaurants with polished businessmen who taught me what foie gras and filet mignon (and receptive oral sex) were. It was because of fatphobic rejection that I didn't end up in an early marriage or feel the pressure of pregnancy like my socially acceptable female classmates whose boyfriends wanted to claim them. It was because I was unencumbered by these things that I could travel and pursue higher education, feminism, and sexual experimentation.

According to the culture, my life mattered less because I wasn't a "fuckable commodity," and so I was pushed to the margins—a glorious and strange borderland, as Gloria Anzaldúa called it. Fatphobia and dieting were like the ghosts that cast a shadow over my life, but as with all oppression it created a road out of the stifling reality of the mainstream. That road is beautiful and amazing, filled with people who know a version of the truth that mainstreamers can't or won't see. I wish everyone had access to that wondrous outcast world, and I wish the terms of that access weren't so barbaric.

I think back on all the things my body sustained at my hands, and how through its refusal to quit or to stop I found my own strength and my own beauty.

Most people cannot even imagine what freedom tastes like, but in my experience it's close to butter. One of the world's favorite fats. For many women I have met, they have lost any appetite for freedom because they have subsisted on so little—both metaphorically and literally—for so long.

What makes freedom difficult is that we have been given no framework to imagine beyond our current state. I once attended a lecture by activist and academic Andrea Smith, who said that in order to accept the unacceptable, we must believe there is no alternative.

I know that when I was in dieting mode I did not think there was any alternative. I believed that it was my job as a fat woman to diet because I had been taught that I needed to change my body by any means necessary. Even though I'm an intelligent, well-read person, it had never even occurred to me that I could opt out of dieting. The thought literally didn't cross my mind until someone introduced it to me in my late twenties—after nearly twenty years of dieting with bouts of starvation. At the time, dieting was as integral to life as air or water. I think I truly believed: I live therefore I diet.

I encourage people to answer this question: What would your life look like if you stopped trying to control your weight?

Let's go further. What would happen if I told you that your body was fine? What if I told you that you have permission to eat whatever you want and wear whatever you want because you are officially perfect? What if we lived in an imaginary world where you had never been taught that your body was wrong, where you never learned that certain foods were good or bad or evil or healthy? What if we lived in an imaginary world where food wasn't charged with any moral meaning—hot dogs weren't morally inferior to carrots, and lettuce wasn't morally superior to Nutella? Imagine that no clothing was off limits—you could wear whatever colors you wanted, stripes that were horizontal or vertical, sequins or chambray, shorts or crop tops. Imagine that every day you woke up and your first thought wasn't "I hate this body." I want you to imagine that you walked around expecting every person to treat you with complete humanity and respect, and when people didn't, you blamed *them* for being assholes instead of blaming yourself for the false perception that you did something to deserve assholery. Imagine that you had never learned that butter was wrong. Imagine that all bodies were seen as equally deserving of affection.

What if I told you that you have the right to that world? What if I told you that you didn't have to lose a pound to earn that life because it was yours at one time, a long time ago, before it was stolen from you?

You Have the Right
to Remain Fat

I wish someone had told me about twenty-eight years ago that it was okay to be fat, that it was, in fact, totally rad to be fat. I wish we lived in a culture where people of all sizes were treated with the full dignity and humanity that each of us deserves.

Almost all of my best experiences and fondest memories have happened around fat people: being raised by two fat women, the way that when I hug another fat person our bellies touch, the first time I went shopping for a two-piece bathing suit, the countless times I have ended up in either a hot tub or an ocean naked, getting breakfast at Eggslut in Los Angeles and then epic chili dogs in Santee Alley where I found a snow-white lace-detailed jumpsuit that reminded me of Selena, that time I peed in a pool at the Marriott in Seattle twice, the plus-size clothing swap where I found a unicorn dress, sneaking onto the set of a music video, going to a party put on by David Lynch, cackling on the side of the freeway while we stared at the moon, eating Puerto Rican plantain-and-steak sandwiches while overlooking the Golden Gate Bridge, learning that the best way to eat popcorn at the movie theater is to sneak in a huge bag of peanut butter M&M's and mix them together, renting a boat to get around the canals just outside of Mexico City while sunning with our rolls out on the wooden deck, the first time I wore a crop top, the time I went to Greece for Orthodox Easter, the time I went and saw a real-life Klimt painting in Vienna, and the time I took a bunch of babes to Jamaica in 2016.

In the fall of 2016 I was in Negril with ten women, most of us fat. I was hosting a retreat for Babecamp, an online course I teach for women who want to break up with diet culture. Each morning we would wake up, eat a huge breakfast of papaya and omelets and pancakes and callaloo and fried plantains and Blue Mountain coffee, then walk down to the white sand beach overlooking the Caribbean Sea to do some meditation, some stretches, and something new I came up with called "jigglecize."

In order to jigglecize you must first decide whether you want to be naked or not. On the first day I decided that in order to get optimal jiggle I would need to take my clothes off. We spread out our arms and legs as far as we could. We dug our bare feet into the warm sand.

I wanted to realize something very old and very playful from inside of us, like the feeling of something ancient being unmoored. I instructed them that I would count down from three and then we would commence shaking every part of us that had any jiggle in it, that we would revel in that delight and curiosity of our bodies the way I had all those years ago when I was a little girl.

Three, two, one . . .

Notes

Restriction Doesn't Work: It's Not You

1. Barbara Boughton, "Obesity a Factor in High-Risk Sexual Behavior in Adolescent Girls," *Medscape*, May 28, 2010, http://www.medscape.com/viewarticle/722673.
2. Michael P. Dentato, "The Minority Stress Perspective," American Psychological Association, April 2012, http://www.apa.org/pi/aids/resources/exchange/2012/04/minority-stress.aspx.
3. Ana Swanson, "What Your New Gym Doesn't Want You to Know," *Washington Post*, January 5, 2016, https://www.washingtonpost.com/news/wonk/wp/2016/01/05/what-your-new-gym-doesnt-want-you-to-know/?utm_term=.881007b9edf9.

Internalized Inferiority and Sexism

1. Emma Gray, "Public Food-Shaming Is the Insidious Type of Street Harassment No One Is Talking About," *Huffington Post*, July 23, 2014, last updated July 1, 2016, http://www.

huffingtonpost.com/2014/07/23/public-food-shaming-women_n_5604185.html.

Fatphobia Is the New Language of Classism and Racism

1. Judy Mandelbaum, "Sex Researchers: 'Size' Does Matter," *Salon*, September 8, 2010, http://www.salon.com/2010/09/08/turkish_sex_study_bmi_male_performance_open2010/. Emphasis my own.
2. Lara Rosenbaum, "4 Exercises That Will Banish Your Man Boobs," *Men's Health*, January 21, 2015, http://www.menshealth.com/fitness/banish-your-man-boobs-0.
3. Angelina R. Sutin, Yannick Stephan, and Antonio Terracciano, "Weight Discrimination and Risk of Mortality," *Psychological Science* 26, no. 11 (2015): 1803–11.

What Early Fat Activism Taught Me

1. Jami McFarland, Vanessa Slothouber, and Allison Taylor, "Tempo-rarily Fat: A Queer Exploration of Fat Time," *Fat Studies* 6 (2007): 1–12.
2. When writing about body positivity, I am referring to the mainstream movement that has arisen as an assimilationist offshoot of the fat liberation movement. There is significant contention among cyberfeminists around what constitutes the "real" body positivity

movement. Some argue that body positivity is
more inclusive and fights for the liberation of
all nonnormative bodies, including not only fat
people but also nonbinary, disabled, and trans
people. Many people who align themselves with
body positivity online (through hashtags, for
instance) still focus primarily on issues of weight
and size (rather than gender or ability). Many of
them are also pro–weight loss and take no clear
stance on their support of fat liberation. Body
positivity has been used as a marketing strategy
by mainstream media and brands. For example,
magazines like *Us Weekly* now write articles
about fat shaming while continuing to glorify
thinness, and plus-size retailer Lane Bryant's
campaign Plus Is Equal (which debuted in 2015
during New York Fashion Week) explicitly
invokes a political ideology to sell clothing. Body
positivity is on the same trajectory as feminism,
shifting from a collective demand for women's
freedom to a simple tagline or commodity.
Mainstream body positivity—with its focus on
feeling positive toward your body rather than
taking concrete steps to end weight-based,
sexist bigotry—leaves much more room for
this "choice feminism" than fat liberation does.
Historically it is this kind of feel-good rhetoric
that facilitates mainstream co-optation and
depoliticization.

Acknowledgments

Thank you to Michelle Tea for encouraging me to write and for giving me a model of existence that I had never imagined before we met. I'd like to thank my past and present editors at the Feminist Press, Jennifer Baumgardner and Alyea Canada. Thank you to Brooke Warner for always giving me no-nonsense advice about all things literary. Thank you to Juliana Delgado Lopera, who encourages me to be honest but also to see the (occasional!) shortsightedness of my own perspective. Thank you to the fat activists and thinkers who came before me and who will come after, who taught me what freedom was and what it could look like—including Charlotte Cooper, Jukie Sunshine, The Fat Underground, Let It All Hang Out, Caleb Luna, Fat Lip Readers Theater, Kendal Blum, It Gets Fatter, NOLOSE, Rachele Teresi,

Nalgona Positivity Pride, Jessamyn Stanley, and Veronika Merklein. Thank you to Isabel Foxen Duke for being a friend and a fellow warrior in this fight for women's lives. Thank you to Sam Tyler-Smith, who I haven't spoken to in years but who changed my life once a long time ago.